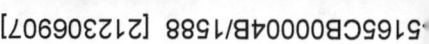

# A Handbook Of Rheumatic Fever

### Dr. Alok Ranjan
MD, DNB, MRCP (UK), DM (Card.)
Sr. Consultant Cardiology
Wockhardt Hospitals
India

authorHOUSE®

*AuthorHouse*™
*1663 Liberty Drive*
*Bloomington, IN 47403*
*www.authorhouse.com*
*Phone: 1-800-839-8640*

*Medicine is a constantly changing science. New research findings necessitate continual changes in disease concept and its management. The author and publisher of this handbook have used reasonable efforts to provide up-to-date, accurate information that is within generally accepted medical standards at the time of publication. However, as medical science is ever evolving, and human error is always possible, the author and publisher (or any other involved parties) do not guarantee total accuracy or comprehensiveness of the information in this handbook, and they are not responsible for omissions, errors, or the results of using this information. The reader should confirm the accuracy of the information in this handbook from other sources. In particular, all drug doses, indications, and contraindications should be confirmed in package inserts.*

*The author has made every effort to trace the copyright holders for borrowed material. If he has inadvertently overlooked any, he will be pleased to make necessary arrangement at the first opportunity.*

*First published by AuthorHouse 09/06/2011*

*ISBN: 978-1-4634-3131-0 (ebk)*
*ISBN: 978-1-4634-3133-4 (sc)*

*Library of Congress Control Number: 2011910950*

*Printed in the United States of America*

*Any people depicted in stock imagery provided by Thinkstock are models, and such images are being used for illustrative purposes only.*
*Certain stock imagery* © *Thinkstock.*

*This book is printed on acid-free paper.*

*Because of the dynamic nature of the Internet, any web addresses or links contained in this book may have changed since publication and may no longer be valid. The views expressed in this work are solely those of the author and do not necessarily reflect the views of the publisher, and the publisher hereby disclaims any responsibility for them.*

Dedicated to my parents; Mr. Bibhuti Bhushan Sinha and Mrs. Rekha Sinha.  I am deeply grateful to their love, care and support for me all my life.

# Table of Contents

# Rheumatic Fever (RF)

Introduction

**Definition**:

Rheumatic fever is expressed as autoimmune **inflammatory** reaction to **collagen fibrils and to the ground substance of connective tissue** leading to **multisystem** involvement and is presumed to be due to antigen mimicry of group A, ß-hemolytic streptococcal pharyngeal infection (GABHS).

RF is the **most common** cause of acquired heart disease in children and young adults worldwide.

## Historical Aspects

Rogers (1910): Noted the **extreme rarity** if not complete absence of RF in India. He observed "Tropical **countries differ in a remarkable way from the temperate in almost complete absence of RF**". Although RF used to be considered a disease of temperate climates, it is now more common in tropical countries, particularly in developing countries

Drury: First ever etiological classification of circulatory diseases in India

Kutumbiah (1935): First Indian doctor to report that rheumatism in childhood was very common in India.

# Incidence and Prevalence

## Incidence

Peak Incidence:    5-15 yrs (School going children)

**< 5 yrs.:**        It is not uncommon to see Acute Rheumatic fever (ARF) in children less than 5 years also. In Indian series up to **40 %** episodes have been documented in less than 5 years of age. The **youngest** age of child reported with ARF is 3 yrs.

## National (India) average

6/1000 (Padmawati et al)
In her series, Delhi recorded the highest incidence of 11/1000 children.

## ICMR (Indian Council of Medical Research):
This study conducted on school children showed higher incidence in urban school children (3.7 – 8 per 1000) as compared to rural school children (3.5 per 1000)

## Prevalence:

Prevalence in Indian population is higher than developed countries

US:  0.6 per 1000

Different studies in India have shown following figures:
Prevalence
Total population
Berry (1972):        1.62/1000
Dhawan/Grover:    0.9/1000

School Children
| | |
|---|---|
| Agarwal: | 0.31 % |
| Padmawati: | 0.15 % |
| Rao: | 0.10 % |
| Devichand: | 3.96 % |

## Reasons for higher and persistently high prevalence in India:

1. Overpopulation
2. Poverty
3. Illiteracy
4. Over crowding
5. Lack of access to medical care
6. Poor compliance (Drop out rate from secondary prophylaxis was 30 %)

# Pathogenesis

Actual pathogenesis of acute rheumatic fever (ARF) remains **hypothetical**. There is **strong but indirect** evidence that Group A Streptococci (GABHS) causes initial and recurrent attacks of RF.

The GABHS infection like any other bacterial infection leads to immune reaction from body. The antibody or cell mediated inflammatory response against GABHS cross reacts with human tissues and leads to development of RF.

The **major factors** that are related to risk of RF are the magnitude of the immune response to the antecedent streptococcal pharyngitis and persistence of organism in throat during convalescence.

## Epidemiology of GABHS infection in relation to RF:

GABHS can cause pharyngitis (rheumatogenic strains), acute glomerulonephritis (nephritogenic strains) or pyoderma (skin strains). The precise factors accounting for rheumatogenicity or nephritogenicity are not known. RF and acute glomerulonephritis (AGN) can occur in same patient and rarely can occur simultaneously also. Although some nephritogenic and skin strains may cause pharyngitis but they do not cause RF. AGN can result from certain rheumatogenic and skin strains.

GABHS pharyngitis attacks spread rapidly due to droplet transmission.

*RF follows tonsillopharangeal infection but **not** infection at other sites

Characteristics of **Etiological agent**:

Group A streptococci (ß - hemolyticus)
Streptococci are rapidly killed by penicillin during mitosis (log phase of growth). Also once phagocytosed by white blood cells, streptococci are highly susceptible to the antibacterial action of oxygen radicals and other antibacterial substances within phagosomes. Therefore, streptococcal infection is primarily **extracellular**, and its **virulence** depends on its resistance to phagocytosis followed by invasiveness and toxin production. Resistance to

phagocytosis is due to presence of capsule and surface M proteins. The hyaluronate capsule resists phagocytosis and internalization of the organism by epithelial cells. It also disrupts connections of epithelial cells and promotes invasion into deeper tissues. The capsule is non antigenic.

Resistance to phagocytosis is further enhanced by several anti-complementary effects of M protein, and by its precipitation of fibrinogen on the bacterial surface. Thus, these 2 factors play an important role in virulence of streptococci. Surface M protein is highly antigenic and induction of type specific anti M antibodies is immunoprotective. However, the multiplicity of M types are responsible for the repetitive nature of GABHS infections and thus for recurrent bouts of RF. Over the period of time, the virulent GABHS strains tend to lose these virulence factors (M protein and capsule). Although, transmission of these attenuated strains lead to high rates of GABHS pharyngitis but the overall incidence of RF decreases. Benign, persistent throat carriage may result from epithelial cell internalization of less encapsulated strains. They may grow more slowly and be less readily eradicated by penicillin.

## Characteristics of **Rheumatogenic** strains of GABHS:

M types 1, 3, 5, 6, 14, 18, 19, 27 and 29
Distinct structural characteristics of M proteins
    Long terminal antigenic domain
    Epitopes that are shared with human heart tissue
Heavily encapsulated, forms mucoid colonies
Resist phagocytosis
Do not produce opacity factor

## Toxins produced by streptococci:

Streptolysin S
    Cell-surface bound hemolysin
    One of the most toxic proteins known (weight by weight)
        Causes rapid destruction of cell membranes
    Very cardiotoxic.

Streptolysin O
  Oxygen labile hemolysin
  Potent cardiac toxin.
Streptokinase
  Liquefies fibrin
Desoxyribonuclease
  Liquefies nucleic proteins
Hyaluronidase
  Promotes rapid spread of the organisms through tissues (e.g., cel-
  lulites and lymphangitis).

Many of these secreted toxins have the properties of superantigens. They
nonspecifically and powerfully stimulate the host's immune response.

## Host Factors:

**Only** humans develop ARF
Genetic predisposition: Familial Tendency: 2 % (India, Padmawati)
  Genetic predisposition is due to
    Presence of specific B cell alloantigen
    High incidence of class II HLA antigen
    • HLA DR 4,21,3,7
      DRW 53, DW 10
      HLA A 19
  Association of HLA antigens has also been demonstrated in Indian
  studies
    Jhinghan et al: Increased frequency of HLA –A33/ D3.
    Decreased incidence of HLA D 2
    Basir Wani (IHJ 1992):
      Increased frequency of HLA DR4 and HLA A 19.
      Significant decrease in B5, B13
**Few characteristics point to presence of other unknown host factors
causing RF**
  Rare before 5 yrs of age.
  Rare in identical twins (about 20 %) than in twins with other immu-
  nological disease such as atopic allergy and hyperthyroidism.
  No clear association with class I HLA antigen
  Definite association with a non HLA B cell antigen

## The inflammatory reaction:

RF develops due to autoimmune reaction against GABHS.
- Cross-reactivity is due to 'antigen-mimicry' (Molecular mimicry)
- The damage to heart is due to **cell-mediated immunity** mediated by T lymphocytes and macrophages.
- Type 2 Hypersensitivity reaction

## Components of GABHS and cross-reactivity with human tissues

| Pathogen | Component | Cross-reactivity |
|---|---|---|
| Capsule | Hyaluronic acid | Joints |
| Cell wall | M Protein/M associated protein | Myocardium |
| Group carbohydrate | N-acetyl glucosamine rhamnose | Valvular tissue |
| Cell membrane | Protein/lipid/Carbohydrate | Myocardial sarcolemma Subthalamic and Caudate nucleus |

# Pathology

The disease process in RF is **diffuse** although the organs mainly involved are heart, joints, brain and cutaneous and subcutaneous tissues. A generalized small vessel **vasculitis** occurs but unlike other vasculitis the thrombotic lesions are not seen. In acute phase of RF, exudative and proliferative inflammatory reactions to connective or collagen tissue occur.

The basic structural change in collagen is fibrinoid degeneration. There is perivascular infiltrate of large cells with polymorphous nuclei and basophilic cytoplasm arranged in rosette around an avascular centre of fibrinoid (**Aschoff nodule or body,** the hallmark of RF). Aschoff bodies are present in any area of myocardium but **not** in other affected organs. They are most often seen in the intraventricular septum, wall of left ventricle or left atrial appendage. Aschoff nodule in proliferative phase is **pathognomonic** of rheumatic carditis. Aschoff bodies are observed in only **30 – 40** % of cases of RF. Its presence is **not** suggestive of recent or active carditis

## Aschoff nodule

Pathognomonic histological lesion seen in RF.
Not seen in first 3-4 weeks of ARF.
Mature Aschoff's nodule is 1 mm to 1 cm in size.
It consists of a perivascular infiltrate of Aschoff's cells and Anitschkow cells arranged in a rosette around an avascular center of fibrinoid. Other cells that can be found in Aschoff body are polymorphonuclear cells and lymphocytes.
Aschoff cell or multinucleate giant cell has 1-5 nuclei and basophilic cytoplasm
Anitschkow cell (cardiac histiocyte or monocyte) is a uninucleate cell with eosinophilic cytoplasm. This cell is normally present in heart but due to active inflammation of ARF, an increase in cytoplasm leads to 'owl-eyed' appearance of the cell.

## Gross pathology seen in RF:

• Acute Rheumatic Fever: Acute Inflammatory Phase

- Heart – Pancarditis
- Joints - Migratory polyarthritis
        Immune complex mediated manifestation
- Skin – Erythema Marginatum
- CNS – Sydenham Chorea

* In Subacute nodule, Erythema marginatum and Chorea: The underlying pathological feature is vasculitis

The acute phase resolves **without** any permanent damage to any organs **except** heart (Rarely, Jaccoud's arthritis may develop)

- Chronic Rheumatic Fever
        Only organ to be affected is heart (Exception Jaccoud's arthritis).
        Characterised by deforming fibrotic valvular disease.

        Progression of valvular stenosis or damage may not entirely be related to recurrent RF infections. Initial alteration in the structure of valve due to valvulitis, changes the blood flow pattern across the valve causing undue hemodynamic trauma to valve. This hemodynamic trauma leads to more fibrosis, thickening and calcification. The rate of progression of fibrosis is higher in patients with more severe initial insult to valve.

        Valve fibrosis and scarring are not specific to RHD can occur after valvulitis (inflammation of all valve layers) due to any cause e.g., RF, brucellar, rickettsial or viral infection. However other infections are very rare in comparison to RF.

        The interval between ARF and development of chronic heart disease in usually 10 – 20 years but this phase is considerably shorter in developing nations.

        The interval between ARF and development of tight MS could be as short as 1 yr (Paul ATS)

Valvulitis due to any cause leads to affection and disruption of all valve layers. The pathological feature is presence of inflammatory cells and vascularisation in all layers. These features are not seen in myxomatous degeneration of valves or other non inflammatory pathologies affecting valves.

# Clinical Features of RF

- Commonest age group: 5-15 years
- Starts as fever with a history of antecedent sore throat (about 2-3 weeks before onset of fever)

## Major Clinical Manifestations: Five

- Polyarthritis
- Carditis
- Sydenham Chorea
- Subcutaneous nodules
- Erythema marginatum

## Joint Manifestations:

Joint symptoms due to ARF are either due to arthritis (major manifestation) or arthralgia (minor manifestation).

## 1. Polyarthritis:

**Most common** (70 %) but **least specific**
Incidence of polyarthritis as seen in **Indian series**

| | |
|---|---|
| Roy et al | 32 % |
| Dhawan/Grover et al | 75 % |
| Agarwal et al | 68 % |
| Sanyal et al | 67 % |

**Definition:**
Polyarthritis is defined as involvement of **2 or more** joints.
Monoarthritis although **unusual,** can occur due to RF.

In Indian series:
Sanyal et al:    Polyarthritis – 87 %;    Monoarthritis - 13 %
Agarwal et al:   Polyarthritis – 93 %;    Monoarthritis – 7 %

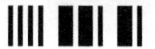

**Pattern of involvement**
    **Sudden onset** with joint pain reaching its peak in 12-24 hours
    **Larger** joints
    Typically involves 5 or more joints
    **Legs first and then spreads to arms.**

The incidence of different joints is as follows:

- Stollerman:
    - Knee                                                                  75 %
    - Ankle                                                                 50 %
    - Wrist, elbow, hip, small joints of legs      12-15 %
    - Shoulder and smaller joints of hands      7-8 %
- Sanyal
    - Knee                                                                  86 %
    - Ankle                                                                 65 %
    - Wrist                                                                 28 %
    - Hip                                                                     15 %
    - Elbow                                                                11 %
    - Shoulder                                                          8 %
    - Uncommon: Spine, metatarsal, temporomandibular, metacorpo-phalangeal and sternoclavicular

**Characteristics of polyarthritis due to RF:**
    It is **almost always**
        asymmetric,
        migratory
            Pain lasts for approximately 1 week in one joint; by the time the joint pain in a particular joint has subsided then the arthritis has migrated to another joint
        involves larger joints.
    Typical clinical features of arthritis are present:
        The joints are swollen, warm, red and tender (minimal redness).
        Patients complain of severe pain and limitation of movements.

**'Pain at rest'** is the characteristic feature

Pain is often **disproportionate** to objective signs (modest swelling and minimal redness)

**Duration of polyarthritis**

Usually resolves within a week (can last for 3-4 weeks) and shows dramatic response to salicylates (within 48 hours). *If there is **no** response to salicylates **within 48 hours** the diagnosis of RF should be questioned.* Rarely some patients do not respond brilliantly to salicylates, requiring supplemental corticosteroids. The arthritis due to RF always resolves with **no permanent damage** to joints except in rare case of Jaccoud's arthritis.

Jaccoud's arthritis

The characteristic deformities of chronic post rheumatic fever arthritis are found in the hand (rarely in feet) and consist of flexion of the metacarpophalangeal joints associated with ulnar deviation of the fingers, most marked in the fourth and fifth digits. The deformities are apparently due to periarticular, fascial, or tendinous fibrosis rather than to synovitis.

This deformity can also affect the feet. Just as the deformity is more marked in the medial digits when the hand is involved, the deformity is most severe in the great toe and the second toe if a foot is affected.

Jaccoud's arthritis is also seen as sequelae to SLE.

**Other arthritic manifestations of streptococcal infection:**

Post Streptococcal Reactive Arthritis (**PSRA**): Arthritis and multisystem involvement following acute streptococcal pharyngitis but
–   Does not fulfill the criteria of ARF;
–   Non – migratory polyarthritis
–   Persistence of arthritis for several months
–   Does not show dramatic response to salicylates;
–   Predilection for females
–   But it should be followed up for subsequent development of carditis. Some PSRA patients apparently have developed rheumatic valvular disease after several years of follow-up (Reported to be as high as 7% of PSRA).

- It is generally agreed to treat PSRA **with the same antibiotic prophylaxis** provided to individuals with RF

**Polyarthralgia:**
>    Joint pains without signs of arthritis.
>    It is considered as **minor** manifestation of RF
>    Must **not** be considered as minor manifestation if arthritis is also present
>    In **Indian series** arthralgia was found to be **more common** than arthritis.

**Incidence:**
>    Roy – 90 %;
>    Padmawati – 46 %.
>    They found "**An inverse relationship between the incidence and severity of carditis and severity of joint involvement**".

## Joint manifestations and incidence of Carditis

| Study | Joint Manifestations | Incidence of Carditis |
|---|---|---|
| Irvington house study | | |
| | Red/hot/painful joints: | 26 % |
| | Tender joints: | 40 % |
| | Joint pains: | 96 % |
| Agarwal et al: | | |
| | Arthralgia: | 100 % |
| | Arthritis: | 45 % |
| Sanyal et al: | | |
| | Arthralgia: | 55 % |
| | Arthritis: | 22 % |

Due to higher incidence and association with more severe carditis, Roy recommended that arthralgia **should** be included as major criteria for diagnosis of RF, should be considered more serious than arthritis and should be treated as aggressively as arthritis for secondary prophylaxis of RF.

## 2. Carditis

- **Most specific** manifestation of RF
- **Pancarditis** (*Affects endocardium, myocardium and pericardium to varying degrees*)
- Incidence: 50 %
    - **Incidence reported in Indian Series**:
        - Sanyal et al:                          33.3 %
        - Grover/Dhawan et al:            37.5 %
        - Roy et al:                              46 %
        - Agarwal et al:                        51 %
        - Abraham/Cherian:          Western: 40-50 %
                                              Developing countries: 64 – 80 %

Rheumatic carditis is **virtually always** associated with the murmurs of valvulitis. Isolated myocarditis or pericarditis without valvulitis is rarely, if ever, due to ARF. So, the diagnosis of valvular involvement is critical and is aided by non-invasive imaging methods. As expected the incidence of carditis is higher if diagnosed by imaging methods.

**Diagnosis**:
Carditis is diagnosed if
**1 or more of the following signs are present**:
a. Significant or new murmur
b. Cardiac enlargement (CE):
More than 15 % increase in cardiac size on standard X-ray (UK and US joint report)
- Pericardial effusion causing CE is **not** included
c. Pericarditis: diagnosed by rub or effusion.
ECG criteria should **not** be taken as evidence of pericarditis **if present alone**
d. Congestive Heart Failure (CHF)

Characteristics:

- Tachycardia during sleep (due to myocarditis) especially in absence of fever and CHF is **reliable sign of carditis**. It is also a **reliable sign for following the course** of carditis

- If present with arthritis: Carditis signs appear within 1-2 weeks of onset of arthritis; **rarely** afterwards

**Murmurs**

- Endocarditis of valve and chordae of Mitral Valve (MV) and Aortic Valve (AV) are characteristic. Tricuspid Valve is involved in about 20 % cases. Pulmonary Valve is almost never involved
- Mitral Regurgitation (MR) is the hallmark of carditis (seen in 90 % cases). Carey Coombs murmur (Mid diastolic murmur) is the flow murmur across MV (of MR). Some authors claim it to be due to valvulitis.
- Aortic Regurgitation (AR): Seen in 20 % cases. AR is usually associated with MR.
- Third heart sound (S3) is often associated with MR.

Pericarditis

- Presence of pericarditis usually indicates pancarditis
    Pericarditis without endo or myocarditis : Think of **etiology other** than RF
- Fibrinous Pericarditis:
    Characteristic naked eye appearance is **'Bread and butter'** appearance
- Incidence:
    - Sanyal et al:        2.9 %
    - Agarwal et al:      13.7 %

Congestive Heart Failure (CHF)

- Incidence : About 5 %
- Indian Series:
    - Sanyal et al:        5.9 %
    - Roy et al:            15 %
    - Agarwal et al:      51.3 %

**Spectrum of Cardiac Involvement in RF:**

- No or questionable carditis

- Definite carditis without pericarditis, cardiac enlargement and failure
- Severe carditis with pericarditis, cardiac enlargement and/or failure

| Incidence | Carditis % | Pericarditis % | CHF % |
|---|---|---|---|
| Massel 1941-55 | 53 | 12 | 15 |
| Feinstein (58-60) | 42 | 7.8 | 13.9 |
| Sanyal (67-71) | 33 | 2.9 | 5.9 |
| Agarwal (80-83) | 51 | 13.7 | 51.0 |
| Bitar (80-85) | 93 | - | 44 |

**Silent Carditis**

- Findings of RHD without history of ARF: Presumed to develop due to an attack of ARF which did not produce CHF, pericarditis or arthritis

- Incidence: 50 % (Stollerman)

**Development of carditis:**
Carditis is usually evident

| Within 1 week: | In 70 % of cases |
|---|---|
| Within 12 weeks: | In 85 % of cases |
| Within 6 months: | In almost 100 % cases |

\* If a patient of ARF **does not** develop carditis **within 6 months**, long term prognosis is excellent if recurrences are prevented

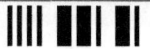

**PR Interval in RF**

- Prolonged
- Reversible
- Does **not** indicate carditis if present alone
- Should **not** be included as minor criteria if carditis is also present
- If present alone, does **not** correlate with the ultimate development of chronic RHD
- This abnormality may be related to localized myocardial inflammation involving the AV node or to vasculitis involving the AV nodal artery.

## 3. *Chorea (Sydenham's chorea / St. Vitus' dance or Chorea minor)*

- Incidence: 20 %
  - **Indian Series:**
    - Sanyal et al:          20 %
    - Roy et al:              5 %
    - Grover/Dhawan et al:    4 %
    - Agarwal et al:          16 %

- **Only** manifestation of RF with sex preference
  - Seen in prepubertal male or females
  - **Never** seen in sexually mature males
  - Increased incidence in pregnancy
- **Delayed** manifestation of RF: appears in 3 months or longer after onset of precipitating streptococcal infection
- Characterized clinically by
  - purposeless and involuntary movements,
  - muscular in-coordination and weakness and
  - emotional labiality

Duration:

Usually resolves in 1-2 weeks but can persist up to 2 yrs.
Chorea most frequently is self-limited but may be alleviated or partially controlled with Phenobarbital or diazepam
Severe chorea seems to respond sometimes to treatment with intravenous IgG.

- Daily handwriting samples can be used as an indicator of progression or resolution of disease
- Benign manifestation

**Differential Diagnosis:**
>Drug reaction (e.g., oral contraceptive pills, phenytoin, haloperidol, amitriptyline, metoclopramide, fluphenazine)
>Huntington chorea
>Chorea gravidum
>Periarteritis nodosa

**Other poststreptococcal movement disorders:**
>Pediatric autoimmune neuropsychiatric disorder associated with *Streptococcus* (PANDAS), and
>Tourette syndrome

## 4. *Subcutaneous Nodules (SN)*

- Incidence:  5 %
  - **Indian Series:**
    - Roy et al:             3 %
    - Sanyal et al:          1.9 %

When present, SN is **mostly seen with carditis** (often multivalvular and severe). In the absence of carditis, the diagnosis of subcutaneous nodules should be questioned.

**Characteristics of SN:**

- Painless, pea size (0.5 – 2.0 cm), firm, freely mobile, occurs in crops
- Overlying skin is freely movable, shows no discoloration and is not inflamed
- Sites:  Extensor surfaces of joints (particularly elbows, knees and wrists), sub occipital region and over spinous processes

Histologically, the SN contains areas resembling the Aschoff bodies observed in the heart.

## 5. Erythema Marginatum (EM)

- Incidence: Less than 5 %
  - Indian series: **Almost never seen**, only 1-2 cases reports are present.

Characteristics of EM:

- Transient (lasts for hours), **erythematous**, macular, **non** pruritic rash with pale centers and rounded or serpiginous margins
- Lesions vary greatly in size
- This characteristic rash is also known as erythema annulare
- Sites: Trunk and proximal extremities,
  - **uncommon** below knee,
  - **Never** on face
- Induced by application of **heat**: Commonly seen after a hot bath and specially after rubbing (drying) with towel

Erythema marginatum has also been reported in association with sepsis, drug reactions, and glomerulonephritis

### Incidence of multiple Major manifestations in a case of RF

Western series:
- Carditis with Polyarthritis:          44 %
- Carditis with Chorea:          14 %
- Carditis with chorea and Arthritis:          6 %
- Arthritis with Chorea:          4 %

### Indian Series

| Carditis with | Sanyal | Grover | Agarwal |
|---|---|---|---|
| Arthritis | 22 % | 29 % | 46 % |
| Arthralgia | 55 % | - | 100 % |
| Chorea | 24 % | - | 25 % |
| SN | 50 % | - | 40 % |
| EM | 100 % | - | - |

## OTHER CLINICAL FEATURES OF RF:

**Fever**
>   Invariably present but rarely more than 39.5° C
>   Continuous and low grade
>   Punctuated by exacerbations, corresponds to involvement of fresh joints or pericarditis
>   Subsides in 3-4 weeks

Epistaxis
>   No diagnostic significance

Abdominal features
>   Abdominal pain
>   Nausea
>   Vomiting

Loss of weight, anemia and fatigue
>   Indicates continuous and **ongoing** disease activity

## Characteristics of clinical features of RF:

### Order of appearance of symptoms of RF

|           | Onset         | Duration        |
|-----------|---------------|-----------------|
| Arthritis | 14 – 35 days  | 3 – 4 weeks     |
| Carditis  | 14 days       | 109 +/- 57 days |
| Chorea    | 2 – 6 months  | 1 wk – 2 yrs    |
| SN        | 1 month       | 8 – 12 weeks    |
| EM        | > 1 month     |                 |

### Duration of Activity of RF

Activity subsides
|                      |                                                  |
|----------------------|--------------------------------------------------|
| Within 6 weeks:      | In 75 % of cases                                 |
| Within 12 weeks:     | In 90 % of cases                                 |
| More than 6 months:  | In Less than 5 % (termed as ***chronic Rheumatic Fever***) |

According to Irvington House Study if ARF lasts more than 223 days (109 + 2 x 57 days) it should be termed as **chronic Rheumatic fever.**

**Resolution of Active Rheumatic fever:**

Activity in RF is considered ended only when both acute phase reactants (ESR/CRP) have become **normal and remain so** for 2 weeks after treatment has been stopped. Occasionally in less than 5 % cases ESR remains high although CRP has become normal, for reasons unknown.

**Developed Vs Developing World**

- In developing countries:
  - More severe with higher incidence of carditis, CHF and mortality
  - EM is never observed
  - Chorea and SN are uncommon
  - Arthralgia is more common
  - Valvular involvement is accelerated and manifests at younger age

    The onset of MS after ARF is very short as compared to western population. Roy et al reported a 2 yr latent period and the shortest period reported is 6 months by Nair et al.

**Characteristics of ARF in Adults**

- Less frequent than children
- Carditis and chorea are less common
  - After 25 yrs., carditis as presenting feature is rare,
    - 14 –17 yrs:     One third (33%) have carditis and
    - < 8 yrs:     90 % have carditis
- EM and SN : Not seen
- Arthritis: More severe, more extensive and lasts longer than children

# Laboratory Investigations

- There are **no** specific laboratory investigations for diagnosis of ARF.

Investigations in RF:

1. Complete blood count
   a. Leucocytosis:
      However, normal count does not rule out ARF.
   b. Anemia:
      Mild to moderate
      Normocytic and normochromic (Anemia of chronic
      inflammatory disease)
   c. High Acute phase reactants –
      CRP, SAA, SAP, Complements, Coagulation Proteins.
      ESR: Typically more than 20mm at 1 hour
      CRP: > 8 mg/dl

2. Evidence of antecedent Streptococcal Infection:
   The best procedure, and one that is used for an acute infection,
   is to take a sample from the infected area for culture, a means of
   growing bacteria artificially in the laboratory. However, cultures
   are useless about two to three weeks after initial infection, so
   Streptococcal antibody tests are used to determine if a streptococcal infection is present.

   Most important investigation to provide supporting evidence of
   antecedent GABHS infection.

   a. Throat Culture:
   b. Streptoccocal antibody tests:
      The commonly used tests are:
         Anti streptolysin O (ASO)
         Anti Deoxyribonuclease B (Anti DNAse B or ADB)
         Streptozyme test (combination of antibodies)
   c. Antigen test

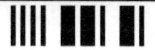

a. Throat Culture:

Rarely positive at the time of diagnosis of ARF.
Positive only in about 11 % of cases.
A positive throat culture or rapid streptococcal antigen test do **NOT** distinguish between recent infection that can be associated with acute RF and chronic pharyngeal carriage of organism. Hence elevated or rising antibody titers are **more** reliable evidence of recent streptococcal infection
Guidelines by expert committees of the American Academy of Pediatrics, the Infectious Disease Society of America, and the American Heart Association favor greater precision in diagnosis by the use of throat cultures.
Throat cultures have the advantage of revealing the presence of mucoid colonies on blood agar.

b. Streptoccocal antibody tests:

80 % of patients of ARF will have raised ASO titers and rest 20 % will have other antibody test positive
When ASO and ADB are performed concurrently, 95% of previous streptococcal infections are detected. If both are repeatedly negative, the likelihood is that the patient's symptoms are not caused by a poststreptococcal disease.
ASO is the recommended test, but when ASO and ADB are done together,
The combination is better than either ASO or ADB alone
Check antibody titers 2 weeks apart to detect a rising titer

1. ASO Titers:
The antistreptolysin O titer, or ASO, is ordered primarily to determine whether a previous group A *Streptococcus* infection has caused a poststreptococcal disease

**Serial increase in ASO titer is more significant**

| | |
|---|---|
| Detectable Level: | Second Week |
| Peak: | 4-6 Weeks |
| Plateau Level: | 3-6 Months |
| Pre Infection Level: | 3-12 Months |

Significant Levels:
     In Children:   **> 333 Todd Units**
     In Adults:     **> 250 Todd Units**

By LATEX Agglutination method: > 200 Units /ml are abnormal

Elevated ASO Antibody levels are also seen in:
    Some healthy children
    Streptococcal C and G infections
    Takayasu's arteritis
    Rheumatoid arthritis
    Henoch Schonlein purpura
False positive tests:
    Hypercholesterolemia,
    Hyperglobulinemia, and
    Liver disorders
False negative tests:
    Antibiotic therapy
    Steroid therapy
    Antibody deficiency syndrome

2.  Anti DNAse B Titer:
    The anti-DNase-B (ADB) test is performed to determine a previous infection of a specific type of *Streptococcus*, group A beta-hemolytic *Streptococcus*

    Abnormal value:
    In children: > 240 Units (Adults > 120)
                      In India > 300 units is abnormal
    **Elevated** even after ASO level becomes normal
    False negative result:
        Hemorrhagic pancreatitis

3.  Streptozyme test
        Detects antibody levels against 5 elements
        Abnormal value: More than 200 units /ml
        Advantages:
            Technically quick and easy
            Unaffected by factors that can produce false-positives
            ASO test

Disadvantages:
    Not as sensitive in children as in adults
    Detects different antibodies, it does not determine which one has been detected
More sensitive but unreliable
WHO has **NOT** recommended it to replace the above 2 tests

c. Antigen test:

Rapid streptococcal antigen test / Rapid Antigen Detection Test (RADT)
    Laboratory confirmation of the presence or absence of GABHS requires throat culture or rapid streptococcal antigen tests. Although in the absence of an immune response, the presence of GABHS by either test is only a presumptive diagnosis (approximately 25% or more may be carriers and thus false positives), *a negative test by either of these methods is a powerful negative predictor of GABHS pharyngitis (>95%)*. Although the *specificity* of some antigen tests has been reported to be as high as 95%, their *sensitivity* may be considerably less. Therefore, when greater precision of diagnosis is critical and the RADT is negative, a throat culture is still recommended.

# Other useful tests in RF:

Rapid detection test for D8/17: This immunofluorescence technique for identifying the B-cell marker D8/17 is positive in 90% of patients with RF, and it may be useful for identifying patients who are at risk of developing RF

Antimyosin antibody imaging: Useful in detecting rheumatic carditis

Cardiac enzymes:
    Are usually low in rheumatic carditis because it is mainly interstitial rather than actual cardiac muscle damage in RF. Troponin 1 levels are low (except when underlying a severe pericarditis). Serum glutamic-oxalacetic transaminase (SGOT) levels are also normal. A raised SGOT level is more likely to be due to salicylate toxicity than due to carditis. The heart failure associated with

acute rheumatic carditis is considered to be due primarily to severe valvular insufficiency, although severe interstitial myocardial inflammation causing myocardial dysfunction has not been entirely excluded as a contributing factor.

Heart reactive antibodies: Tropomyosin is elevated in persons with acute RF

**X-ray chest**
> Cardiomegaly
> Signs of cardiac failure
> *A normal CXR does not exclude the presence of carditis*

**ECG:**
> Sinus Tachycardia
> Conduction defects (45 – 70 %)
>> Prolonged PR
>> 2nd degree AV block
>> Complete and high grade AV dissociation: Rare
> Signs of myocarditis and pericarditis
>> In individuals with acute pericarditis, ST segment elevation may be present, most marked in leads II, III, aVF, and $V_4$ through $V_6$
> Dysarrhythmias

**Echocardiography:**

Echo-Doppler examination in more sensitive than clinical examination in detecting carditis in ARF and can contribute to early and definitive diagnosis and better prophylaxis. As valvulitis is the most common manifestation of carditis and so the finding of valvular involvement is critical and is aided by echo-Doppler studies. Echo-Doppler is even more helpful in subauscultatory cases. Eltohami et al found in their study that carditis was identified clinically in 43 % and with addition of echocardiography in 71 % of cases. Clinical examination may also over diagnose rheumatic carditis. In a study, only 40.6 % of clinically diagnosed carditis was proved on echocardiography and in remaining 59.4 % carditis was ruled out by echo study. The murmurs in these cases were due to functional murmur, congenital heart disease and other causes. Echo is useful in detecting carditis in some high risk group like patients with chorea and silent carditis. Echocardiography probably has a better place in developed countries where incidence of ARF is very low and severe carditis is unlikely. Prognostically, absence of carditis on echocardiography may indicate good long term prognosis.

It is now important to include results from recent long term studies, to establish more precisely the natural history of the subauscultatory rheumatic valvular regurgitation as diagnosed by echocardiography. Such information will influence the choice and duration of secondary prophylaxis.

## Echo feature of RF

MV / AV thickness > 4 mm
MR grade > I – II
Mitral Valve prolapse (MVP)
Rheumatic nodules (beaded appearance)
AR
TR
Pancarditis
Pericardial effusion
Chordal tear

## Right Ventricular Endomyocardial Biopsy

The yield of useful additional clinical information from endomyocardial biopsy (EB) has been low.

Its diagnostic sensitivity in one relatively large study was only 27%. In patients with chronic rheumatic heart disease, however, EB does not appear to provide additional diagnostic information.

In patients with rheumatic carditis EB should be limited to clinical investigation.

# Diagnosis of RF

There is **no specific** clinical, laboratory or other test that establishes the diagnosis of RF.

Diagnosis is based on criteria proposed by T Duckett Jones. Several amendments have been done to increase its utility.

- Proposed by T Duckett Jones:     1944
- Modified Jones criteria:          1956
- Revised Jones criteria:           1965
- Amended Jones criteria:
- Updated Jones criteria:           1992

**Jones Criteria of Diagnosis:  Updated 1992**

- **Major Criteria**
  - Polyarthritis
  - Carditis
  - Subcutaneous nodules
  - Erythema marginatum
  - Sydenham Chorea

  **Remember "JONES'**
  - **J**: Joints
  - **O**: ♡
  - **N**: Nodule
  - **E**: Erythema marginatum
  - **S**: Sydenham Chorea

- **Minor Criteria**
  - Clinical features
    - Fever
    - Arthralgia
  - Elevated Acute phase reactants
    - ESR/CRP
  - Prolonged PR interval on ECG

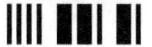

**Evidence of antecedent GABHS infection:**
> Positive throat culture or rapid streptococcal antigen tests or high or rising streptococcal antibody titer

**Presumptive Diagnosis of ARF**
> If supported by evidence of preceding GABHS infection, the presence of
> **Two Major** or
> **One major and two minor criteria**
> indicates a **high probability** of acute rheumatic fever

**Amended Jones criteria**
- Suggested by Roy, Massel
- Supported by Agarwal and Cherian
- Useful for developing countries.
    - Erythema marginatum should be dropped from major manifestations' list
    - Arthralgia with high ESR and high ASO titer ($\geq$ 400 Todd units) should be made a major criteria
    - Evidence of preceding streptococcal sore throat should be made a minor criteria and not mandatory for diagnosis

**Exceptions to Jones Criteria**
> Most patients with recurrent ARF also fulfill the Jones criteria, but in some the diagnosis of a recurrence is less obvious.

- Three notable exceptions to strict adherence to the Jones criteria
    1. Chorea: It may occur late and be the only manifestation of RF.
    2. Indolent carditis: Patients presenting late to medical attention, months after the onset of RF and may have insufficient support to fulfill the criteria.
    3. Newly ill patients with a history of RF, especially RHD, who have **supporting evidence of a recent GABHS infection** and who manifest either a single major or several minor criteria. A presumptive diagnosis of rheumatic recurrence may be made in these cases; distinguishing recurrent carditis from preexisting significant RHD may be impossible.
        When rheumatic valvular disease pre-exists, clear recognition of a new bout of carditis requires evidence of fresh cardiac injury

such as pericarditis, acute cardiac enlargement and/or congestive heart failure, or a newly detected murmur from a valve not previously affected.

The Jones Criteria, therefore, apply more readily to initial attacks, and more diagnostic latitude is sometimes needed to interpret recurrent carditis in patients with pre-existing rheumatic heart disease

## Problems with the Diagnosis of RF

A definite diagnosis of RF is important since it commits an individual to prolonged prophylactic antibiotic therapy. Moreover, the diagnosis of RF may be particularly difficult when there is only one major manifestation. Unfortunately, RF remains a clinical syndrome **without** a single pathognomic feature. The Jones criteria became particularly useful in clinical investigation. Thus, these guidelines avoid overdiagnosis but do not always establish the more subtle manifestations of the disease.

Adding evidence of antecedent GABHS infection helps in detecting cases of RF particularly in presence of single major manifestation.

Isolated polyarthritis:

The diagnosis of isolated polyarthritis is problematic because of the large differential diagnosis. However, polyarthitis appears early in the rheumatic attack when streptococcal antibodies are at peak elevation. Therefore, the absence of significantly increased GABHS antibodies at the onset of polyarthritis is a useful negative factor of the diagnosis of ARF and suggests a reactive arthritis due to another infection, such as rubella, Lyme disease, the enteric organisms causing Reiters disease, ankylosing spondylitis, etc. When GABHS antibodies are increased, however, the diagnosis of ARF in isolated cases of polyarthritis remains presumptive, requiring months of close observation because such elevations may have been only coincidental GABHS infections not causally related.

Chronicity of the arthritis, and particularly its recurrence in the absence of a new GABHS pharyngeal infection, the appearance of joint deformity, or the presence of rheumatoid factor or ANA antibodies may eventually reveal a different disease, (e.g. rheumatoid arthritis, systemic lupus, polyarteritis, etc.). Although typically migratory, this feature may not be present in all cases. Hence 'polyarthritis' rather than 'migratory polyarthritis' is considered as major criteria in Jones criteria. Polyarthritis may be additive rather than migratory, particularly in initial phase. It may persist in many joints at once, and furthermore stubbornly "rebounding" once or twice after six week courses of anti-rheumatic therapy.

## Isolated Chorea and Post-Infectious Autoimmune Neurological Diseases (PANDAS)

PANDAS are often associated with antecedent GABHS infection and some cases have clearly been shown to be associated with deposition of streptococcal antigens in the basal ganglia.

PANDAS might well be included, like PSRA, as variable features of the syndrome of ARF.   Currently, the role of GABHS pharyngitis as a cause of recurrent episodes of obsessive-compulsive disorders in children without chorea or other PANDA manifestations is being evaluated.

## Isolated carditis:

The finding of valvular involvement is critical to the diagnosis of rheumatic carditis and is much aided by non-invasive imaging methods. (See; Echocardiography)

# Treatment

*Primary Prevention* of Rheumatic Fever

**RF is a complication only of GABHS pharyngitis.** Prevention of RF therefore depends on either the prevention or proper treatment of GABHS pharyngitis.

All cases of suspected streptococcal pharyngitis should be treated aggressively to prevent ARF.

**Differential diagnosis with viral pharyngitis is required but may not be possible in all cases.**

The most common cause of sore throat and upper respiratory tract infection is viral infection. GABHS pharyngitis needs to be differentiated from it. The presence of fever, chills, toxic appearance, exudative pharyngitis and tonsillitis with enlarged cervical lymph nodes favor GABHS and presence of cough, rhinorrhoea, viremia (bodyache, malaise and fever) and hoarseness favor viral infection. However adenovirus and infectious mononucleosis may cause exudative lesions and some GABHS strains may cause non exudative sore throat. In such cases only laboratory investigations can help to differentiate between the two.

**Treatment of an acute attack of GABHS pharyngitis.**

Ideally, treatment of GABHS sore throat should be started promptly. However, delay of a few days while awaiting culture results does not interfere with primary prevention of ARF

Antibiotics:

Group A streptococci are uniformly highly sensitive to penicillin. (penicillin resistant GABHS strains have not emerged)

Benzathine benzylpenicillin:

Single IM injection

Dose:
> For children less than 30 kg body weight
>> 600,000 IU
> For cases more than 30 kg body weight
>> 12, 00,000 IU

Mixtures of benzathine benzylpenicillin with procaine benzylpenicillin G have been used. The mixture tends to cause less discomfort, but doses must be calculated based upon the amount of benzathine benzylpenicillin in the mixture
Rate of fatal anaphylaxis:  1:10,000 cases

Phenoxymethylpenicillin (Penicillin V)
> Oral for 10 days
> Dose:
>> < 30 kg: 250 mg 2 or 3 times daily
>> > 30 kg: 500 mg 2 or 3 times daily

A 10 days course of treatment is required
> 10 day course of oral penicillin is more effective than 7 or 5 days course of oral penicillin in achieving bacteriological treatment and prevention.  10 days course ensures maximum eradication of bacteria.
> To minimize diarrhea associated with oral antibiotics, it is recommended that penicillin should be taken with 2-3 tablespoonful of yogurt or with lactobacillus tablets.

For penicillin allergic patients:
> Erythromycin ethylsuccinate
>> Oral for 10 days
>> Dose:  40 mg/kg/day (max. 1.5 g/day) in 3 divided doses
> Erythromycin estolate
>> Oral for 10 days
>> Dose:  20 - 40 mg/kg/day (max. 1.5 g/day) in 3 divided doses

Alternative treatment:
1) Oral ampicillin or amoxicillin has been used. They must be given for 10 days.
2) Oral cefalosporins (first or second generation) are also effective but usually are more expensive.  They must be given for 10 days

3) Newer orally administered macrolides have been reported to be effective in eradicating GABHS when given for less than 10 days. At this time data are not sufficiently conclusive to support unqualified recommendation for a shortened course of therapy.
4) Despite these alternative treatments, penicillin remains the drug of choice because of its proven efficacy in preventing rheumatic attacks, its low cost, and its relatively narrow antibacterial spectrum
5) Sulfonamides or tetracycline are **not** acceptable therapy for GABHS pharyngitis
6) Antibiotic regimens that produce *total* eradication of GABHS pharyngeal carriage are not required. GABHS strains persisting following adequate therapy are usually attenuated, so that follow-up cultures and retreatment of asymptomatic patients with persistent throat carriage is not required.
7) GAS carriage is difficult to eradicate with conventional penicillin therapy. Thus, oral clindamycin (20 mg/kg/d PO in 3 divided doses for 10 d) is recommended

**"Mass" Primary Prophylaxis of RF in Epidemics**
May be required
Such events are now rare now except in military populations or in closed institutions.
A single injection of 1.2 million units of benzathine penicillin G administered to each person in affected population.

# Treatment of ARF

**Treatment remains supportive.**

1. Primary prevention of GABHS pharyngitis should **always** be given to eradicate any existing bacteria.

2. Bed Rest:
   **Absolutely necessary.**
   It should be continued till fever abates or till acute phase reactants have decreased to normal values.

   *Recommended period of rest is:*
   Arthritis alone:         2 weeks
   Carditis:
        Uncomplicated:      4 weeks
        With cardiomegaly:      8 weeks
        With CHF:      8 weeks or till failure is controlled

3. Medications:

a. **Aspirin (acetyl salicylic acid -325 mg)**
   100 mg/kg/day in divided doses for 2 Wks (Max. dose: 4 – 6 gm/day)
   60 mg/kg/day in divided doses for next 6-10 Wks
   Attempt to keep aspirin blood levels from 20-25 mg/dl, but stable levels may be difficult to achieve during the inflammatory phase because of variable GI absorption of the drug.
   Maintain aspirin at anti-inflammatory doses until the signs and symptoms of acute RF are resolved or residing (6-8 wk) and the acute phase reactants (APRs) have returned to normal.
   Average duration of treatment: 6-12 weeks

   Slowly taper and discontinue in a week or two: When discontinuing therapy, withdraw aspirin gradually over weeks while monitoring the APRs for evidence of rebound.
   Watch for salicylate toxicity

Side effects:
  Gastritis and acid peptic disease (Watch for black stools).
  Ototoxicity
  Hyperventilation
  Metabolic acidosis

Other NSAIDs can be used to treat ARF:

**Ibuprofen**
  Dose:  Children over 6 months of age is 7-10 mg / kg every 6 hours
  Avoid this drug in children with liver, kidney, stomach or bleeding problems.
**Naproxen**
  Dose for children > 13 yrs is 10-20 mg / kg / day BD with food.  Max dose 500 mg per day.
  Avoid this drug in children with liver, kidney, stomach or bleeding problems.

The **new COX-2 inhibiting NSAIDs**, though expensive, may reduce the adverse effects of large doses of aspirin.

**b.  Corticosteroids**:

  Indications:-
    CHF,
    Cardiomegaly, and
    Pericardial effusion
  Steroids should be given with aspirin to provide maximum benefit. As the dose of steroids is tapered, dose of aspirin should be increased and it should be continued after stopping steroids to prevent rebounds of RF.

  Dose schedule:
    Initial 2 -3 weeks:
      Prednisolone:  1 mg /kg/day (Max.  60 mg/day)
      Aspirin: 40 mg /kg/day
    After 2 -3 weeks:
      Prednisolone:  Should be tapered gradually and discontinued in 4 –5 weeks.  Taper 20-25% each week

Aspirin: Should be increased to 50 – 60 mg / kg / day and continued for 6 weeks following withdrawal of prednisolone.

Important points:

- Prednisolone should be given in single dose and with milk. Antacids should be added to minimize acidity and gastritis.
- Therapy of ARF does **not** provide any **prognostic** benefit, i.e., it does not decrease the chance of future development of RHD.
  **Treatment of RF remains supportive**.
  Steroids do **not** prevent valvular damage
  The more potent anti inflammatory effects of steroids are justified only in severe carditis (with CHF). In such patients the powerful suppression of inflammation may at times make management easier by suppressing fever and reducing toxicity and anemia.
- **Only** prevention of further attacks of ARF can **decrease** the chance of chronic valvular heart disease
- Rebounds are frequent following steroid withdrawal
- Mild rebound should not be treated aggressively.
- Steroids rapidly controls acute manifestations but is **not** superior to salicylates except in severe carditis

## Newer Treatment of RF

IV gamma globulin
No effect on course of illness. May be effective in severe chorea.
Anti-TNF drugs: Under trial
Because valvular scarring is suspected to be the result of cytotoxic cellular autoimmunity, anti-TNF drugs that delay or reduce joint destruction in rheumatoid synovitis may deserve a trial in severe acute rheumatic carditis to determine whether they might similarly reduce valvular injury and scarring.

## TREATMENT OF CHF

Complete bed rest
Steroids: Must as it reduces mortality
Diuretics
ACE inhibitors

**Mortality of ARF:**
    Depends on severity of carditis
        Indian series:
            Sanyal:             0.98 %
            Agarwal:          2 %

**Treatment of severe carditis and outcome**

Massell et al (N = 137)

| | Improved | Death |
|---|---|---|
| No Rx (n=40) | 36 % | 47 % |
| Aspirin (n=42) | 43 % | 21 % |
| Steroids (n=53) | 92 % | 4 % |

Probably, early and effective control of inflammation in steroid arm is responsible for low mortality.

# Recurrences Vs Rebounds of RF

Differentiation between these two is based on:

1. Preceding streptococcal infection
2. Symptom free period of 3 Months
3. APRs: ESR and CRP

Rebounds: Defined as
- Reappearance of clinical features and acute phase reactants
- Increase in ESR; CRP remains **normal**
- Not preceded by streptococcal infection
- Rebounds occur within 2 months of cessation of treatment and are most common in first 2 weeks.

**Importance of CRP**
- Reflects rheumatic activity more closely than ESR;
- Unaffected by anemia, changes in serum proteins, and heart failure
- Useful in confirming rebounds

**Characteristics of recurrence of RF:**
Recurrences are common
Incidence of recurrence depends on following factors:

- Time since last attack of RF:

|  | Rate of recurrence |
|---|---|
| − Within 1st yr: | 50 – 65 % |
| − 1 - 5 yrs: | 11 – 23 % |
| − 5 –10 yrs: | 4.8 % |

- Chemoprophylaxis era
  - IM prophylaxis: 1 in 250 patient years
  - Oral prophylaxis: 1 in 25 patient years

- Prechemoprophylaxis era
  - 1/5 in 5 yrs
  - 1/10 in 5 – 10 yrs

- Age of patient:
  - Younger the patient : Higher the recurrence rate
    1 in 4 if age < 9 yrs
    1 in 8 if age > 16 yrs

- Increased antibody response (High titers) to streptococcal infection: Higher value is associated with higher recurrence rate

- Epidemic Vs endemic infection

|  | Recurrence rate |
| --- | --- |
| Epidemic | 3 % |
| Endemic | 0.3 % |

- Related to symptomatic severity of pharyngitis (Irvington house study)

|  | Recurrence rate |
| --- | --- |
| – Asymptomatic infection: | 10.3 % |
| – Infection with fever and sore throat: | 31.7 % |

- Related to severity of established disease

|  | Recurrence rate |
| --- | --- |
| – RF with no RHD: | 10 % |
| – RF with RHD: | 27 % |
| – RF + RHD + CE + CCF: | 43 % |

- **Recurrence tends to mimic prior episodes in 90 % cases:** Hence if carditis was absent in first attack it is likely to be absent in subsequent attacks of RF.

- Latent period of rheumatic fever does **not** get shorter in recurrence

**Difference of Clinical Features between First Attack and Recurrence**

|  | First Attack | Recurrence |
|---|---|---|
| Valvulitis | New onset of SM, Carey Coombs, AR | Change in murmur New onset of murmur |
| Myocarditis | Unexplained cardiomegaly Unexplained CHF/Gallop sounds | Worsening of CE Worsening of CHF. |

## Initial attack of ARF and evolution of RHD:

After first attack of ARF, even if subsequent attacks are prevented by adequate penidura prophylaxis there is still risk of development of RHD. The risk of RHD is high if carditis was present in the first attack. If there is recurrence of RF, the risk of development of RHD is very high. Hence the recurrences of RF should be prevented aggressively.

| ARF | Development of RHD | No RHD |
|---|---|---|
| Without Carditis | 8 % | 92 % |
| With Carditis | 66 % | 34 % |

Hence, after an attack of ARF, even if subsequent attacks of RF are prevented there is still 8 % chance to develop RHD. As evident in the table the risk is substantially higher with carditis. In patients who had carditis, development of RHD is also linked with severity of carditis.

## Initial attack of ARF and evolution of RHD: With Carditis

| With Carditis | Development of RHD | No RHD |
|---|---|---|
| Without CHF or pericarditis |  |  |
| Mild MR | 33 % | 67 % |
| Moderate MR | 65 % | 35 % |
| Severe MR | 80 % | 20 % |
| With CHF and / or Pericarditis | 86 % | 14 % |

Hence, with severe carditis (with congestive heart failure and pericarditis) 86 % of cases will ultimately develop RHD and only a small group (14 %) may not develop any residual heart disease if subsequent attacks of RF are prevented.

# Secondary Prevention of RF

Benzathine benzylpenicillin:  IM Injections
  Dose:
    For children <30 kg body weight:  600,000 IU every 3-4 weeks
    For children > 30 kg and adults:  1,200,000 IU every 3-4 weeks

Phenoxymethylpenicillin:  Oral
  Dose:  250 mg 2 times daily

Sulfonamide (e.g. sulfadiazine, sulfadoxine or equivalent):  Oral
  Dose:
    < 30 kg: 500 mg daily
    > 30 kg: 1.0 g daily

Erythromycin:  Oral
  Dose:  250 mg 2 times daily

Recurrence in Post Chemoprophylaxis Era
  • IM Penicillin:      0.4 per 100 pt. Yrs
  • Oral Penicillin:    4 per 100 pt. Yrs
  • Sulfadiazine:       2.8 per 100 pt. Yrs

Oral penicillin is the least effective of all regimens.

Incidence of recurrence in different series:

U.K. and U.S. Joint Report (n=369) 1951-52
  5 yrs:              2.3/100 Patient yrs.
  10 yrs:             2/100 Patient yrs

Feinstein et al (n=431) 1954-60
  5-6 yrs:            2.9/100 Patient yrs

Sanyal et al (n=65) 1967-71
  5 yrs:              0.6/100 Patient yrs

Lue et al (n=131) 1961-75
  5.5 yrs:                    1.68/100 Patient yrs

**Duration of secondary prophylaxis:**
  WHO Recommendations
      Patients with No carditis or RHD:
          Up to 18 years of age and at least five years after the last attack
          of RF, whichever is later.
      Patients with documented carditis:
          At least to 25 years of age or 10 yrs since last attack of RF,
          whichever is later.
      Patients with Chronic carditis:
          For life
      Patients with artificial valves:
          For life

**Secondary prevention of RF:**
  Benzathine penicillin every three weeks (In areas where RF is very
      prevalent)
  Ensure that the commercial formulation employed contains the full
      dose of 1.2 million units of benzthine penicillin G and not con-
      fusing formulations that contain smaller amounts of benzathine
      penicillin G mixed with shorter-acting penicillin G compounds.
  The quality of the vehicle ensuring good suspension of the particles of
      this poorly soluble penicillin salt is also important to ensure the
      uniform delivery of a proper dose. Available preparations may not
      be of uniform quality in all parts of the world.
  Oral prophylactic regimens are also effective but are less reliable. They
      are recommended when the risk of rheumatic recurrences is rela-
      tively low.
  Oral penicillin is the least effective and also leads to emergence of
      alpha streptococcus. It may cause Infective endocarditis. Hence
      it should also be remembered that while treating IE in a patient
      who are already on penicillin prophylaxis, penicillin agents should
      not be used for treating IE

**Duration of secondary prophylaxis** for rheumatic subjects depends on a
  number of variables that influence the rate of recurrences.
      Presence or absence of rheumatic heart disease,

The time elapsed from the previous attack,

The number of previous attacks, and

The severity of the antecedent infection.

Variation in the local prevalence of rheumatogenic streptococci.

In areas of the world where rheumatic fever is still frequent, patients with rheumatic heart disease may have to be maintained on prophylaxis indefinitely. On the other hand, prophylaxis has been safely stopped after several years of treatment when rheumatogenic streptococci have been shown to have disappeared from a community. For patients without rheumatic heart disease, the duration of prophylaxis may be shortened to approximately five years, depending again on the risk of exposure to GABHS pharyngitis in cohorts and to the prevailing epidemiology of RF.

In India also, in a large study from Vellore, the recurrences of RF were found to be significantly low after 26 years of age. Hence duration of secondary prophylaxis can be modified with lesser risk of infection.

**Risk of Recurrent Infection and duration of secondary prophylaxis:**

| Category | Risk of recurrence | | |
|---|---|---|---|
| | **High** | **Not high** | |
| | | Age < 40 yr | Age > 40 yr |
| RHD | Life long | Till 40 yrs of age | None |
| ARF with carditis but without RHD | Till 40 yrs of age | 21 yrs of age or 10 yrs since last attack | None |
| ARF without carditis | Till 21 yrs of age or 10 yrs since last attack | 21 yrs of age or 5 yrs since last attack | None |

## Infective Endocarditis (IE) prophylaxis in a case of RHD

Do not use penicillin, ampicillin, or amoxicillin for endocarditis prophylaxis in patients already receiving penicillin for secondary RF prophylaxis (relative resistance of oral streptococci to penicillin and aminopenicillins due to chronic penidure prophylaxis). Alternate drugs recommended by the American Heart Association for these patients include oral clindamycin (children: 20 mg/kg; adults: 600 mg) and oral azithromycin or clarithromycin (children: 15 mg/kg; adults: 500 mg).

Antibiotic regimens used to prevent recurrences of ARF are inadequate for prevention of IE

Patients who have had RF but there is no RHD do not need IE prophylaxis

# Future

Prospects of A Vaccine Against Rheumatic Fever

Because immunity to GABHS is type specific and dependent on antibodies to M protein, attempts at vaccine production have focused primarily on M protein purification. An effective vaccine against rheumatic fever may not require the inclusion of all known M protein serotypes, but rather those identified most clearly as containing rheumatogenic strains. A recombinant, multivalent vaccine containing the type-specific epitopes of some 26 M serotypes associated the great majority of serious GABHS infections is currently under field trial. The potential for the production of IgA antibodies to M proteins by employing such preparations for oral human immunization is suggested by recent experimental studies. The protective role of mucosal IgA and its production by oral streptococcal vaccines is under vigorous current investigation.

Vaccines are under trial that may lead to protection against the most virulent and dangerous of known GABHS strains.

# Recommended Reading

1. Stollerman GH. Rheumatic fever and streptococcal infection. In: Stollerman GH, ed. New York: Grune & Stratton, 1975
2. Rowe JC, Bland EF, Sprague HB, White PD. The course of mitral stenosis without surgery: ten and twenty years perspective. Ann Intern Med 1960;52:741-749
3. Olesen KH. The natural history of 271 patients with mitral stenosis under medical treatment. Br Heart J 1962;24:349-357
4. Sanyal SK, Thapar MK, Ahmed SH, Hooja V, Tewari P. The initial attack of acute rheumatic fever during childhood in North India: a prospective study of the clinical profile. Circ 1974;49:7-12.
5. Sanyal SK, Berry AM, Duggal S, Hooja V, Ghosh S. Sequelae of the initial attack of acute rheumatic fever in children from North India: a prospective 5-year follow up study. Circ 1982;65:375-379
6. Roy SB, Bhatia ML, Lazaro EJ, Ramalingaswami V. Juvenile mitral stenosis in India. Lancet 1963; 2:1193-1196
7. Roy SB, Gopinath N. Mitral stenosis. Circ 1968;38(Suppl V):68-76.

# Abbreviations

ACE: Angiotensin converting enzyme
AGN: acute glomerulonephritis
Anti DNAse B: Anti Deoxyribonuclease B
APR: Acute phase reactants
AR: Aortic Regurgitation
ARF: Acute Rheumatic Fever
ASO: Anti streptolysin O
AV: Aortic Valve
AV block: Atrio-ventricular block
AV dissociation: Atrio-ventricular dissociation

CCF: Congestive cardiac failure
CE: Cardiac enlargement
CHF: Congestive heart failure
CNS: Central nervous system
CRP: C reactive protein
CXR: Chest X-ray

EB: Endomyocardial biopsy
ECG: Electrocardiogram
EM: Erythema Marginatum
ESR: Erythrocyte sedimentation rate

GABHS: Group A, ß-hemolytic streptococcus

HLA: Human leucocyte antigen

IE: Infective endocarditis
IgA: Immunoglobulin A
IgG: Immunoglobulin G
IHJ: Indian Heart Journal
IM: Intra-muscular
IU: International Units
IV: Intra-venous

MR: Mitral Regurgitation
MV: Mitral Valve
MVP: Mitral Valve prolapse

NSAID: Non steroidal anti-inflammatory drug

PANDAS: Pediatric autoimmune neuropsychiatric disorder associated with Streptococcus
PSRA: Post Streptococcal Reactive Arthritis

RF: Rheumatic Fever
RHD: Rheumatic heart disease
Rx: Treatment

S3: Third heart sound
SAA: Serum Amyloid A
SAP: Serum Amyloid P-component
SLE: Systemic lupus erythematous
SGOT: Serum glutamic-oxalacetic transaminase
SM: Systolic murmur
SN: Subcutaneous Nodules

TNF: Tumor Necrosis Factor
TR: Tricuspid Regurgitation

WHO: World Health Organization